Live Better shiatsu

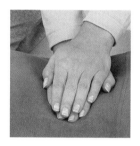

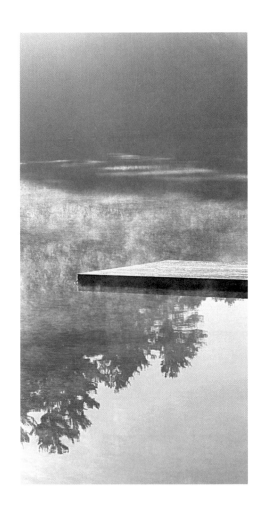

Live Better shiatsu

exercises and inspirations for well-being

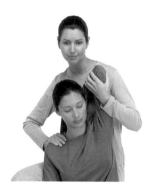

Chris Jarmey

DUNCAN BAIRD PUBLISHERS

LONDON

Live Better: Shiatsu

Chris Jarmey

First published in the United Kingdom
and Ireland in 2005 by
Duncan Baird Publishers Ltd
Sixth Floor, Castle House
75–76 Wells Street, London W1T 3QH

Conceived, created and designed by
Duncan Baird Publishers Ltd
Copyright © Duncan Baird Publishers 2005
Text copyright © Chris Jarmey 2005
Commissioned artwork copyright © Duncan
Baird Publishers 2005
Commissioned photography copyright ©
Duncan Baird Publishers 2005
For copyright of agency photographs see p.128,
which is to be regarded as an extension of this
copyright.

The right of Chris Jarmey to be identified as
the Author of this text has been asserted in
accordance with the Copyright, Designs and
Patents Act of 1988.

Managing Designer: Manisha Patel
Designer: Justin Ford
Managing Editor: Grace Cheetham
Editor: Rebecca Miles
Picture Research: Julia Ruxton
Commissioned Photography: Matthew Ward
Commissioned Artwork: Debbie Maizels

British Library Cataloguing-in-Publication Data:
A CIP record for this book is available from the
British Library.

ISBN: 978-1-84483-238-5

10 9 8 7 6 5 4 3 2

Typeset in Filosofia and Son Kern
Colour reproduction by Scanhouse, Malaysia
Printed by Imago, Malaysia

Publisher's note

Please note that this book is not intended
as a "teach yourself" manual and is no
substitute for professional training. Before
following any advice or practice suggested
in this book, it is recommended that you
consult your doctor as to its suitability,
especially if you suffer from any health
problems or special conditions. The
publishers, author and photographers
cannot accept any responsibility for any
injuries or damage incurred as a result of
following any of the advice or exercises in
this book, or of using any of the therapeutic
techniques described or mentioned here.

contents

INTRODUCTION

The pace of life today is rapid, and it seems to be getting ever faster. At one time the majority of interpersonal communication was face to face. Now many of us are just as likely to text or email other people instead. Of course, modern technology is not all bad – it frees up our lives in many ways and enables us to expand our horizons – but it has led to us living in an era of more messages and less conversation, more crowding and less real contact.

To me, real contact is the fundamental issue. Looking into someone's eyes and actually talking to them conveys so much more than a miniature screen full of acronyms without punctuation. And what about real physical contact? People are well connected through cyberspace, but how much better is a hug, or at least a handshake? We humans are social animals who need physical contact, and direct social interaction. These are some of the basic reasons why people love to receive bodywork of all kinds. It is a form of caring touch that feels good and leaves the receiver with an ongoing sense of well-being.

Shiatsu is a bodywork system from Japan that has two distinct realms of application: the amateur and the professional. In Japan there is an amateur in almost every household who gives shiatsu from time to time to other members of the family, to ease out the stresses and stiffness resulting from everyday life. There are also professional therapists who you can visit if there is a more serious medical problem. Whether you have an amateur shiatsu or a professional treatment, one common factor is that it feels absolutely great to receive. People visit shiatsu professionals not only to resolve health issues; they also go for the sheer pleasure of it.

In this book we explore the history and theories behind shiatsu, learn about its benefits and techniques of application, and see how these are put together to form basic shiatsu sequences that are highly beneficial to general health. In the West we are still a long way from having an amateur shiatsu practitioner in every house, but with this book I hope to encourage a greater awareness and appreciation of the practice of shiatsu, and to promote the study and application of this healing art.

HOW TO USE THIS BOOK

Shiatsu is a versatile system of bodywork that can be practised at many levels. This book provides practical information and examples for you to refer to if you are learning basic-level shiatsu, or if you simply wish to discover more about this increasingly popular and widespread therapy. However, it is not intended to be a "teach yourself" manual. Rather you should use this book to supplement a shiatsu training course. It will help you to remember how to perform and apply basic shiatsu techniques. It also offers a concise guide to the theories behind and benefits of shiatsu for ready reference. For information on finding reputable shiatsu practitioners and training establishments, see p.128.

Different levels of shiatsu practice

This book is most appropriate for those interested in beginner-level shiatsu – the type that is suitable to practise on family and friends for the purpose of de-stressing them and boosting their immune systems.

This level requires a good grasp of shiatsu techniques, and training in how to stay relaxed and comfortable as you work. A thorough foundation course of around 12 to 14 days will offer sufficient training to achieve this, assuming you practise your skills between classes. For this reason a course spread over a few months is better than an intensive period of study, because it gives plenty of opportunity to practise what you learn at each stage.

If you are interested in taking shiatsu further and becoming a professional therapist, you will need around three years of training to reach a suitable level and gain the level of touch sensitivity and confidence required for professional practice. The Shiatsu Society, a governing body for the profession, requires three years of study and practice before entering a graduate on its register.

There is also an intermediate level, where you can qualify in Japanese Bodywork after one year of shiatsu training. This level is called *Anma-Sotai*, and includes shiatsu for muscular, joint and postural problems only, rather than the full range of diagnostic and treatment skills learned by a fully-qualified shiatsu therapist.

origins and basics

Shiatsu is a method of bodywork based on traditional Oriental philosophy and medicine, which has at its core a belief that everything in existence is a manifestation of energy. This universal energy, called Ki (sometimes spelled Qi or Ch'i), needs to flow around the human body smoothly in order that the body can maintain optimum health and help prevent illness. Ki links all the functions and organs of the body through a system of interconnecting channels (sometimes called meridians). Each Ki channel flows both near the surface of the body and deep inside it to connect with the internal organs. All of the Ki channels are connected to form a continuous circuit of Ki flow, animating all parts of the body as it passes through. The ultimate aim of shiatsu is to keep the Ki flowing without restriction, and the Ki channel sections near the surface of the body are the parts that are accessible to shiatsu technique.

In this chapter we begin by looking at the specific psychological focus required for successful shiatsu practice. We then learn something of shiatsu's historical background and how the practice has evolved into its present forms. We examine the theories behind and the benefits of shiatsu, look at its links with other therapies, and assess the importance of the correct working environment for shiatsu work.

THE SHIATSU MIND

The literal translation of the Japanese word *shiatsu* is "finger pressure", although the practice involves far more than simply applying pressure with the fingers to someone's body. The fundamental principle of shiatsu is to hold, with clear mental focus, sustained stationary contact with a person's body. Practitioners do this by using thumbs, fingers, palms or sometimes forearms, elbows or knees, with sufficient patience to wait for a response in the receiver's subtle flow of life-sustaining vitality (Ki). A variety of stretching, rotating and levering techniques may be required to reduce the receiver's muscular and mental tensions, but essentially, the giver uses stationary pressure at the appropriate angle and depth. This is what differentiates shiatsu from massage.

Shiatsu demands an ability on the part of the practitioner to focus the mind in order to detect subtle changes within the receiver's Ki. As such it requires a high level of humility and skill in order to assist the natural healing process without superimposing personal expectations on the situation. Shiatsu works more deeply if we understand that we cannot help restore true health effectively if we fail to acknowledge and respond to the person's own life energies. Professional shiatsu practitioners spend many years in training, learning to listen to those energies and assist their natural inclination toward balance and harmony. One core shiatsu aim is, therefore, to nurture the potential for revitalization of both the receiver's body and their mind.

The shiatsu therapist's mind is trained to focus solely on the present, and to empty itself of both preconceptions and expectations. To be fully aware of the present moment is the only way the practitioner can truly empathize with the receiver, and give them the best possible treatment as a result. In shiatsu we aspire to keep our consciousness fully in the present for as much of the session as possible. Most methods of meditation have the same purpose. In this sense shiatsu is as much a practice for developing self-awareness as it is a physical therapy. It is not so much mechanically physical, but rather physically mindful.

HISTORICAL BACKGROUND

Shiatsu was first developed in Japan in the 1920s. It evolved from older forms of Chinese bodywork that are still practised today. The blanket term for traditional Chinese bodywork is *An Mo* (*Anma* or *Amma* in Japanese). *An Mo* literally means "press" (*An*) and "rub" (*Mo*). It has four major branches, each one defined by its own specialized techniques. These are *Pu Tong An Mo* (general massage), *Tui Na An Mo* ("push-grab" method), *Dian Xue An Mo* ("cavity press" method) and *Qi An Mo* (Ki method). All *An Mo* is based on the principles of traditional Oriental medicine. The degree to which shiatsu incorporates these principles varies according to the style of shiatsu practised.

In the early 20th century, Oriental medicine was generally discouraged throughout Japan in favour of Western medicine. This was reflected in the way that many leading *Anma* exponents abandoned their Oriental medicine heritage. However, not all Japanese bodyworkers accepted this trend toward stripping away the base of traditional theory and practice in their work. These practitioners, along with many of their contemporaries in acupuncture, worked toward re-establishing Oriental medicine as their theory base and, in the 1920s, changed the name of their practice to shiatsu.

After the Second World War, the proportion of classic Oriental medicine utilized within shiatsu once again declined, giving way to a greater emphasis on Western medical theories. Although the predominant style of shiatsu in Japan today is still based mostly on Western medicine, the latter part of the 20th century saw an increased reintegration of traditional Oriental medicine into many styles of shiatsu; particularly those now commonly practised in the West. Whichever style of shiatsu is practised, all share many fundamental principles of how to apply pressure and stretch. All styles have some techniques influenced by modern Western osteopathic or chiropractic methods, particularly those concerned with muscle lengthening, and mobilizing joints. Today, shiatsu continues to grow and develop, as its Oriental medicine base is explored ever more deeply.

SHIATSU STYLES TODAY

Over the years shiatsu has developed various nuances in the way in which it can be applied. Today, in both Japan and the Western world, shiatsu practitioners perform several different categories or styles of shiatsu, each of which emphasizes one or more of these nuances, without ever loosing the basic principle of applying direct pressure to the receiver's body. The main styles are:

1 **Acupressure shiatsu** This focuses upon techniques where pressure is applied to specific points on the body to initiate a predetermined effect. It is basically acupuncture without needles.

2 **Five Element shiatsu** This focuses primarily on an aspect of Oriental medicine known as Five Elements, or Five Phases. These elements or phases reflect the various cyclical phases of nature as observed throughout the year. Such phases are also seen as having parallels within the human body and mind. So, human rhythms and cycles reflect, and are in tune with, the broader phases

of the environment. Treatment using the Five Element method is about harmonizing the patient's own cycles of vitality with nature's seasons and cycles.

3 **Macrobiotic shiatsu** This follows the philosophy of balancing body and mind by eating foods considered to harmonize rather than stimulate or suppress vitality. Shiatsu in this context is used to help support the energetic harmony derived from the patient's specific diet and lifestyle.

4 **Nippon shiatsu or Namikoshi method** This places more emphasis on Western physiological explanations about shiatsu's effects, and minimizes its reliance on traditional Oriental medicine theory. It is a style currently very widespread within Japan.

5 **Zen shiatsu** Developed by Shizuto Masunaga in the 1970s, this style uses an extended system of Ki channels and an amalgam of Oriental medicine theory, Western medical physiology and Western psychology.

6 **Ohashiatsu** Broadly speaking this is an amalgam of Nippon and Zen styles. It was developed and propagated by US-based Japanese practitioner Wataru Ohashi.

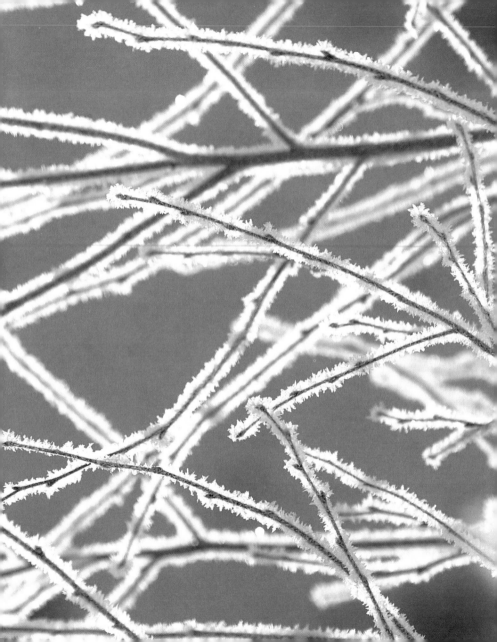

All things are connected,
like the blood which unites one family.
All things are connected.
Whatever befalls the earth befalls the sons of the earth.

CHIEF SEATTLE

(c. 1790–1866)

SHIATSU AND OTHER THERAPIES

Shiatsu is sometimes confused with other therapies and can be misrepresented as a result. It does, however, have close links with other bodywork systems, some of which can support and complement its techniques very well.

Shiatsu is often mistaken for massage, and, indeed, both practices can be considered bodywork. However, massage implies kneading, squeezing and rubbing the soft tissues of the body to benefit those tissues, whereas shiatsu focuses on applying direct pressure to the body and stretching the limbs – it addresses the rebalancing of Ki more than the detoxification or toning of physical tissues; although, clearly, one influences the other. Also, normally massage is applied directly on to bare skin, whereas shiatsu is given through a layer of clothing.

Japanese *Anma* therapy (see p.14) is much closer to what we would recognize as massage. In fact both *Anma* and Swedish massage have their roots in older bodywork methods that originated in China. However, *Anma* is also a precursor of shiatsu in that most of the original shiatsu practitioners started out as *Anma* therapists.

In terms of theory, shiatsu is most closely linked to acupuncture as both practices share the same theoretical roots in Oriental medicine and both aim to affect the body's Ki distribution directly. Acupressure has some similarities with shiatsu because it, too, is concerned with affecting certain points on the body via touch. However, shiatsu has a broader range as it employs various stretching and manipulation techniques as well as sustained touch. Acupressure methods are often incorporated as a subdivision of shiatsu.

Some see parallels between shiatsu and reflexology, but although reflexology uses direct thumb pressure on a body-part, it is based on an entirely different theoretical model. However, both disciplines combine well.

Hands-off or light-touch healing methods, such as reiki, have some similarities with an aspect of specialized shiatsu known as "etheric work". This is work upon the receiver's "Ki field" which makes no actual physical contact. Similarly, etheric shiatsu is very similar to what is known as medical Qigong, or Qigong healing.

THE BENEFITS OF SHIATSU

Shiatsu work will benefit absolutely anybody who receives it because it seeks to promote a balance and harmony within your body's energy and we are all out of balance at some level. Either we have too much pent-up energy in some areas of our bodies and minds, and/or we lack vitality in other areas. By helping to regulate our bodies' Ki, shiatsu helps to restore this balance.

You do not have to be ill to receive shiatsu. Treatment will help to maintain existing good health, and can also act as a preventative against illness. However, if you are suffering from an ailment, shiatsu can usually help in many ways by aiding the creation and support of an optimum bodily environment in which the body can heal itself. Even the most basic shiatsu is able to calm you if you are stressed, or loosen up your tense muscles and stiff joints. It will also improve your general level of vitality by boosting your circulation and your immune system. The list opposite gives some examples of the general benefits of shiatsu work.

Shiatsu helps to:

- increase energy levels
- increase body awareness
- relieve stress-related anxiety and tension
- induce deep relaxation
- ease aches and pains
- boost the immune system
- fight common ailments
- increase flexibility
- heal sports and dance injuries
- stabilize emotional and psychological conditions
- relieve backache
- improve posture
- improve stamina
- improve digestion
- improve libido
- treat menstrual problems
- support a healthy pregnancy
- ease childbirth
- relieve headaches and migraines
- harmonize body, mind and spirit

CONTRAINDICATIONS

Young, old, frail, strong – if you can be touched, you can receive shiatsu. However, there are some circumstances where it is inappropriate for a shiatsu practitioner to give treatment, or it may be limited in its effectiveness, purely because touch is difficult at that time. The following list highlights some contraindications for shiatsu.

Acute fevers Most of us prefer to be left alone when we are aching and sweating from a fever.

Contagious diseases Do not give shiatsu to someone suffering from a disease that can be acquired through touch because of the risk of cross-infection.

Severe skin problems Avoid giving shiatsu if a receiver is suffering from a skin condition that renders physical touch painful – it could also be damaging to the affected area of skin.

Bone, muscle or ligament injury Do not apply shiatsu to swollen areas, fracture sites or areas where there is acute muscle or ligament injury.

Internal bleeding or blood clots If the practitioner has any suspicion of internal bleeding or blood clots in the receiver they should avoid giving shiatsu because it encourages an increase in blood flow. Also, blood clots are likely to break up or dislodge when pressed, or if blood flow is markedly increased.

Varicose veins Avoid direct presssure on varicose veins as it is likely to aggravate them. However, shiatsu given elsewhere on the body may help the condition.

Pregnancy Shiatsu can be both highly relaxing and invigorating during pregnancy. However, work on certain pressure points (such as many on the lower leg) can increase the risk of miscarriage. It is safest to avoid giving shiatsu to pregnant women altogether unless you are a specially trained and experienced professional.

Basically, if you have trained properly (see pp.8–9), follow a common-sense approach, and take into account these contraindications listed above, you can practice shiatsu safely on other people in order to boost their Ki and prevent the potential onset of disease.

THE IDEAL WORKING ENVIRONMENT

The environment in which you practise shiatsu plays a vital part in its sucessful application. Here we describe how to ensure optimum working conditions for the benefit of both the practitioner and the receiver.

One of the advantages of shiatsu is that it requires no specialized equipment, other than a mat and a couple of cushions. As a result, it is a very portable form of bodywork. However, most professional shiatsu practitioners will rent a room in their local complementary medicine clinic. Some also work in specialized hospital clinics. Others may visit the receiver's place of work or residence. Many practitioners also convert a room in their own home specifically for giving shiatsu. Those who practise only basic shiatsu techniques on friends and family, will usually give shiatsu at the recipient's home, or use a room in their own house.

Wherever you give shiatsu, it is extremely important to do everything possible to encourage within yourself a greater equanimity of mind and a clear mental focus before working. As far as possible avoid situations that are likely to place you under stress immediately prior to practising shiatsu. For example, if you have to travel, make sure you leave plenty of time to reach your destination – worrying that you are running late is not the best preparation for shiatsu work.

You cannot always choose where to give shiatsu, but if you are in a position to select the optimum location and can influence the ambience of the room, then the following suggestions will be useful.

The ambience of your shiatsu room

Setting aside a dedicated room solely for shiatsu is the ideal. This is because the feeling and ambience experienced within a defined space, especially an enclosed space, will gradually become influenced by the activities that take place there. For example, if a room is used mainly for bitter arguments, then a "bitter argument" atmosphere will permeate the feel of that room. Conversely, if the room is used solely for shiatsu and activities that prepare you for giving shiatsu (such as meditation and yoga), it will take on the same peaceful atmosphere associated with shiatsu itself.

Creating an ambience of peace and serenity in a room has many clear advantages. First, those who receive shiatsu in that room will react by starting to relax even before you begin working on them. Much of the preparatory work toward reducing their stress and tension at the beginning of a session will have been fulfilled by the room itself. Second, when the positive ambience of the room builds to a sufficient level, the space will become like a sanctuary for you. You will find that upon entering the room to give shiatsu, the familiar feeling of serenity associated with that activity in that particular space will override any negative feelings you may have at that time. For example, if you have been working downstairs on a stressful project, upon entering your "sanctuary" you will soon feel as if all that is far away. You will in effect have entered a bubble that seems divorced from the normal stresses of life.

If you cannot reserve a whole room for shiatsu, try to allocate a space within a quiet room, normally used for

THE IDEAL WORKING ENVIRONMENT

activities that are not too frenetic or depressing. A good
ambience will still begin to manifest there, but maybe
not so quickly or strongly. If you cannot reserve a corner
solely for shiatsu, at least try to give shiatsu in the same
place each time. Just going to that familiar location will
trigger your mind to switch into shiatsu mode.

The contents of your shiatsu room

Keep your shiatsu space as free from clutter as possible.
All you need is a mat about 2 metres (6ft) in length by
1.5 metres (4½ft) wide, with enough room around it to
apply your shiatsu. A professional shiatsu practitioner
will usually use a shiatsu futon, which is a mat consisting
of two or three layers of compressed cotton or wool,
contained within a cotton covering. The futon would be
between 2.5 and 4 cm (1 and 1½in) in depth, compressing down a little with use. For hygiene place a cotton
sheet over the futon and provide a small cloth or some
soft paper about the size of a pillowcase to place under
the receiver's head, particularly if they are in the face-
down position. Have three or four fairly firm cushions

nearby so that you can support the receiver's head and limbs when required.

Lying in a cold room is not much fun for the receiver, so be sure to keep the room warm. In addition provide a blanket to keep him or her especially cosy once you have finished work. You may also like to use a lightweight cloth about $70cm^2$–$1m^2$ (2–$3ft^2$) to place between the receiver's skin and your hands when working on areas such as their neck or face, particularly if their skin is sweaty or greasy.

The shiatsu space must be as neutral as possible, free from metaphors relating to your personality. You could have some attractive plants and perhaps a few soothing pictures on the walls to enhance the calm feeling of the room, but keep it simple. You might interpret these suggestions as a restriction to the expression of your personality, and may want to include art and décor that reflects the inner "you". But reflecting "you" is not the point in this particular room. You have the rest of your house for that. Remember, this room should be a sanctuary, a place totally removed from the rest of daily life.

Appropriate clothing

Many bodywork therapies are delivered on to the unclothed patient. Shiatsu, however, is usually applied through a layer of clothing. This is because the sensory nerve endings are most prolific on the skin, and skin-on-skin contact distracts the giver from feeling the deeper, subtle presence of Ki. Clothing acts as a barrier to dampen down the surface tactile sensations felt by both the giver and receiver. As a result, both people are able to experience a deeper connection to the Ki that lies just below the surface.

Both the giver and receiver of shiatsu will benefit from wearing loose-fitting clothing that enables maximum movement of the limbs. Cotton clothing works better than synthetic fibres because synthetic fibres seem to interfere with the flow of Ki. Also, the practitioner should avoid wearing any items of clothing, such as belts or untucked shirts, that might inadvertently brush against the receiver during treatment, as this can be very distracting. Basically your clothing should be clean, comfortable and functional.

Tension is who you think you should be.

Relaxation is who you are.

CHINESE PROVERB

Let the beauty of what you love be what you do.

RUMI

(1207–1273)

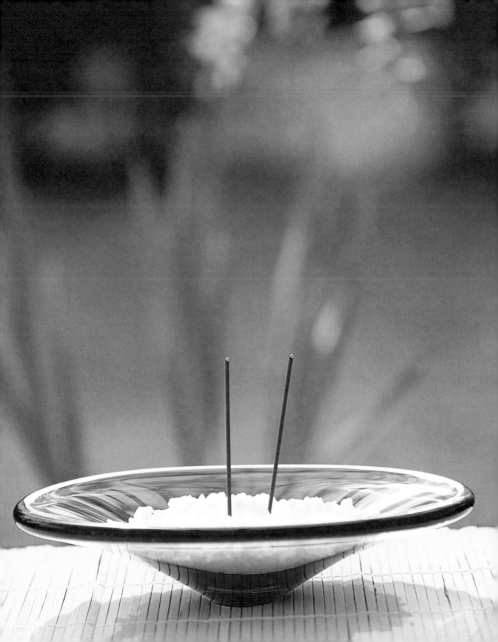

Chapter Two

the body in balance

Shiatsu is placed firmly within the broader context of
traditional Oriental medicine, and anyone wishing to
learn about shiatsu or, indeed, become a shiatsu
practitioner should be acquainted with the theories
upon which Oriental medicine is based. This holistic
and comprehensive system of medicine is a vast sub-
ject and takes years of study to understand fully.
However, a knowledge of its workings is vital for professional shiatsu practitioners if they are to be able to
appreciate their patients' needs and to formulate
appropriate treatment strategies.

In this chapter we explore some of the basic con-
cepts that underpin the traditional theories of

Oriental medicine that are relevant to professional shiatsu practice, with a view to gaining a general appreciation of the logic and simplicity, yet profundity of this ancient system of understanding the body and mind. We start by looking at the philosophy of Yin and Yang, which links all things in the universe and gives us great insight into how the health and vitality of humankind is influenced by the energies, forces and rhythms of the universe in which we live. We discuss the manipulation of the body's Ki by shiatsu work on the different Ki channels and we learn about *kyo* and *jitsu*, the two opposing states that can affect the flow of Ki around the body.

YIN AND YANG

One of the most fundamental philosophies behind traditional Oriental medicine is the principle of Yin and Yang. Yin and Yang are opposite but complementary forces that exist within everything in the universe. They must co-exist in a balanced state to regulate harmony throughout our bodies and our minds.

Yin-Yang theory states that all things consist of two opposite forces that struggle against one another and keep one another in check. For example, cold cools down heat – this is why cooling drinks refresh on a hot day. Equally, heat warms up cold, which is why a fire will warm you on a cold day. Aiming for a balanced and harmonious interaction between Yin and Yang is the basis of all treatment in Oriental medicine. For example, if you have a hot condition, such as a fever, treatment should be cooling, and vice versa.

Yin and Yang are wholly interdependent and neither can exist in isolation. Their characteristics are often represented by opposing pairs by way of explanation.

Thus, Yin and Yang can be seen as cool and warm; shade and sunlight; night and day; winter and summer; material and immaterial; internal and external; earthly and heavenly; feminine and masculine; structure and function; body and mind; *kyo* and *jitsu*; loose and tense.

Another feature of Yin and Yang is that they tend to consume one another. This means that where Yin predominates it will overwhelm and use up Yang, and vice versa. For example, for the body to work normally and keep itself warm (Yang), it has to burn up part of its substance (Yin). On the other hand, ingesting and processing nutrients (Yin) consumes a bit of energy (Yang).

Yin and Yang can also transform into each other. The cycle of day transforming into night and back to day, and the yearly seasonal cycles are examples of this. Finally, every phenomenon can be divided into Yin and Yang over and over again an infinite number of times. Hence within autumn, the beginning will be more Yang (closer to summertime) and the latter part will be more Yin (closer to wintertime). The latter half of autumn can be divided yet again in the same way and so on.

KI, *TSUBOS* AND CHANNELS

The universal energy known as Ki flows around the body along a series of interconnecting channels, many of which have been identified by Oriental medicine practitioners over the centuries. Fourteen of these channels contain pressure points that directly influence the body's organs and their associated functions, and these are the channels on which professional shiatsu practitioners focus during treatment.

At specific locations along the Ki channels, there are special "gateways" where Ki can access or leave the body via a point on the body's surface, the skin. These gateways are known as *tsubos* and, when touched by a shiatsu practitioner, they provide crucial information concerning the regulation of the flow of Ki around the receiver's body. Also, the practitioner's technique of touching and stretching the body can "activate" the *tsubo* and cause it to affect positively both the channel of Ki in which it is located and this channel's associated organs and body/mind functions.

A *tsubo* is like a vortex of Ki that, if you could see it, would resemble a vase-shaped swirl of energy with its mouth at the surface of the body, leading into a slender neck, widening into a broader belly below the surface.

Each of the 14 primary channels (see pp.40–41) has a number of "fixed" *tsubos*, each of which has a name, number and recognized action on the body when stimulated by shiatsu work. In addition to the fixed *tsubos*, there are "transient" *tsubos*, which appear and disappear along the channels between the fixed *tsubos*. These arise where and when they do because there is either a lack of Ki or an excessive build up of Ki at that particular location and at that particular time along the channel. Where Ki is lacking, the *tsubo* will feel lifeless and empty. It may feel stiff and lifeless or flaccid and lifeless. Where Ki is blocked and consequently overcrowded, there will be a feeling of fullness, tightness and constriction at that location, often accompanied by pain if touched.

Shiatsu focuses on methods to re-balance Ki via the *tsubos*. The techniques and sequences shown later in this book illustrate some of the different ways to do this.

Shiatsu work is holistic and supports the idea that body and mind are wholly interconnected. Students of shiatsu learn how each Ki channel corresponds to different aspects of the mind and emotions as well as to parts of the physical body. For example, the liver influences our ability to make good plans yet remain flexible

THE FOURTEEN MAIN CHANNELS OF SHIATSU

The channels are shown here on three separate diagrams. They are drawn on one side of the body only although apart from the Governor Vessel and the Conception Vessel (which run down the centre), each channel is reflected in an identical position on the other side of the body.

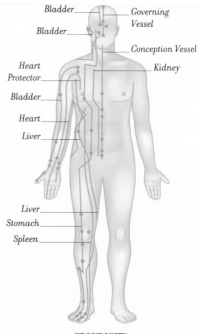

FRONT VIEW

enough to change direction if the original plan fails. Likewise, it ensures flexibility of body by ensuring a smooth flow of Ki and nourishment to our tendons, ligaments and muscle fibres. Each part of the body has similar links or "correspondences" to other mental and emotional activities in the same way.

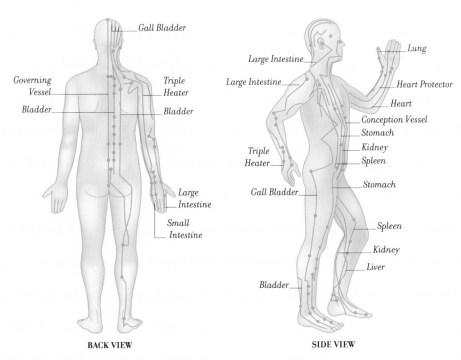

BACK VIEW   **SIDE VIEW**

KYO AND JITSU

In shiatsu terminology weakness or emptiness of Ki is referred to as *kyo* whereas fullness or blockage of Ki in a channel or *tsubo* is known as *jitsu*. You can expect any channel to err toward *kyo* or *jitsu* in relation to any other. The whole pattern throughout the body is constantly fluctuating. The aim of shiatsu is to discover the root cause behind any acute or chronic disharmony in a person's Ki and to attempt to stabilize it. This is achieved by the manipulation of the affected area, and is known as the "tonification" of the *kyo* or the "dispersal" of the *jitsu* within the channels. (For further explanation of tonification and dispersal of Ki in shiatsu, see pp.58–9.) The *jitsu* areas are easy to find because they feel "active" and may protrude from the surface. *Kyo* areas are more difficult to locate because they exhibit little or no reaction, and are hidden below the surface.

Sensitive shiatsu performed all over the body will highlight these *kyo* or *jitsu* deviations and re-harmonize the general level and flow of Ki. However, an experienced professional practitioner would also be able to assess which channel is most lacking in Ki, and which one is most blocked, and tailor treatment accordingly. Because all of the Ki channels in the body flow into one another to form a continuous circuit, by working to balance out *kyo*-heavy and *jitsu*-heavy channels the shiatsu practitioner will also be helping the receiver's body to regulate lesser imbalances in its other channels.

It takes many years of shiatsu practice to be able to properly identify and assess levels of *kyo* and *jitsu* in someone's Ki channels. Much imbalance can be subtle and difficult to detect, but it is imperative to be confident in any diagnosis, as incorrect treatment can have the opposite effect to the one we desire. Ultimately you are aiming for the harmonization of Ki and creation of the optimum conditions for the receiver's body and mind to achieve the best health they can.

For additional reference the table presented on the following pages outlines some of the clear comparisons that exist between the states of *kyo* and *jitsu* within the Ki channels of the human body.

Kyo

- Represents a need, which requires the Ki to be strengthened

- Indicates an underlying cause

- Is an empty state that requires filling

- Indicates stagnation in the channel owing to the lack of Ki being unable to sustain enough momentum for Ki circulation

- Is an underactive state, leading to flaccidity or stiffness

- Is found below the surface

- Is less obvious

- Is slower to respond to treatment

- Requires deep, sustained connection

- Is treated by tonification, which affects the whole person

Jitsu

- Represents the body's attempt to restore harmonious Ki flow

- Manifests as symptoms

- Is a full state that requires emptying or dispersing

- Indicates stagnation in the channel owing to too much Ki occupying a confined area (like a traffic jam)

- Is a hyperactive state, leading to congestion and blockage

- Is found protruding from the surface

- Is more obvious

- Usually responds immediately to treatment

- Requires a moving technique or to be left alone

- Is treated by dispersal, which affects localized body areas

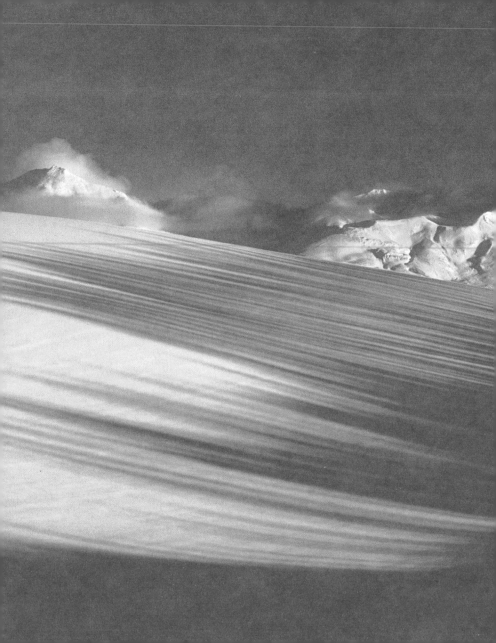

I am the dust in the sunlight, I am the ball of the sun ...
I am the mist of the moraine, the breath of evening ...
The rose and the nightingale drunk with its fragrance.
I am the chain of being, the circle of the spheres,
The scale of creation, the rise and the fall.
I am what is and what is not ...
I am the soul in all.

RUMI

(1207–1273)

Chapter Three

shiatsu techniques

Before describing how shiatsu skills are developed, it is important to reflect on the benefits that can be obtained from its practise. The purposes of giving shiatsu to your friends and family-members are primarily to help them to relax and combat stress. This, in turn, will help improve their circulation of blood, lymph and vitality (Ki), thereby boosting their immune system. Furthermore, shiatsu is generally effective for alleviating stiffness and aches and pains throughout the body. It also helps both the giver and receiver become more aware of their bodies, and encourages the development of healing compassion through appropriate physical contact.

This chapter describes how to administer the various shiatsu techniques to optimum effect. We begin by examining the seven qualities practitioners need to develop in order to fully hone their skills. We then look at the importance of correct posture for the giver and correct position for the receiver during a treatment session. This is followed by a comprehensive description of how to apply the various "tools" of shiatsu, in other words how different parts of the body, such as the fingers, thumbs, elbows, knees and feet, can be used to apply pressure or a stretch. Finally, there is a concise description of the theory behind efficient shiatsu stretching methods.

THE PRACTITIONER'S APPROACH

There are seven qualities that are generally accepted in shiatsu circles as being essential for developing a good prefessional technique. Without these qualities, shiatsu is a more mechanical and less profound practice; ultimately less effective and resulting in a less enjoyable treatment for the receiver.

1 **Motivation** Shiatsu will definitely be more enjoyable and effective (for both practitioner and receiver) if you are truly motivated to help other people to feel better. It seems to be universally believed that the more you give of yourself in the service of other people, the more the universal energy of Ki will come flooding back to you. So if you are strongly motivated to help others you will also be helping yourself.

2 **Steadiness of breath** If you breathe deeply, in a relaxed way, your mind will become steady, and you will become "centred". Shallow, irregular breathing, by contrast, will render your thoughts scattered and unfocused. This

illustrates the close connection between the breath and the thought processes. By steadying the breath and, therefore, the mind, the giver of shiatsu will be able to feel more of the subtle fluctuations in tension within the receiver. This will result in a deeper and more effective shiatsu treatment.

3 **A strong and open *hara*** In common with the Japanese martial arts, shiatsu gives great emphasis to ensuring that all movements originate from the central pivotal area of the body. This is centred in the belly, or *hara* as it is called in Japan. For example, when using the thumb to apply pressure, the shiatsu practitioner is trained to be aware that the movement starts from the *hara*. By constantly focusing the mind in the *hara*, energy becomes focused there, resulting in greater harmony of body, mind and spirit. This awareness should help the practitioner to relax their *hara* while giving shiatsu, which improves balance and helps release tension.

4 **Comfort and relaxation** If there is tension in your body or mind when you give shiatsu, it is usually felt by the recipient, who will often duplicate that tension within

their own body and mind as a result. Ensuring that you assume and maintain a good position that is free from strain is of great importance in order to attain the correct physical and, therefore, emotional equilibrium necessary for effective shiatsu practice.

5 **"Empty mind" state** Having established the correct motivation, breathing and body position, shiatsu should be applied through feeling rather than thinking. It is a physiological fact that the less we think about something the more we can feel. This is because our intuition (associated with right-brain activity) is suppressed if too much thinking (associated with left-brain activity) is happening and vice-versa. In shiatsu we call this non-thinking attribute "empty mind". So, we use our thinking process before and after the session to diagnose and evaluate the condition of the receiver, but employ our intuitive "empty mind" state to feel more during the hands-on phase of the session.

6 **Offer support to the receiver rather than force** This has several meanings. First, we can provide support through offering a sympathetic attitude to any of the

receiver's physical or emotional problems. Second, we can actively support their physical position, with cushions where appropriate, to ensure their maximum stability during a session. Third, we can offer a supportive touch when applying shiatsu techniques, so that we lean into the receiver with gravitational pressure rather than push or shove them. And finally, we can be available to offer a supportive and reassuring word or two at the end of the treatment session.

7   **Competent technical ability** This refers to the shiatsu practitioner having a comprehensive range of techniques on which to draw. All of these need to be applied appropriately and without effort; with fluency of movement and empathy of spirit.

If you learn about, understand and, above all, seek to emulate these seven qualities, you will be taking great strides toward achieving the correct technical, physical and emotional approach required of all shiatsu practitioners, and as a result your shiatsu sessions will yield immense benefits to those receiving treatment.

CORRECT POSTURE AND BODY POSITION

It is particularly important to be mindful of your posture when giving shiatsu, because poor postural alignment will result in you experiencing discomfort and fatigue, especially if you are giving several shiatsu sessions in a row. Where you position yourself in relation to the receiver will also have a bearing upon your comfort. If you are not comfortable you will end up concentrating more upon your own aches and pains and less upon the person to whom you are giving the treatment.

The use of *hara*

Shiatsu technique should never come from muscular strength, but should utilize gravity wherever possible – always lean rather than push or pull. To lean correctly, we need to be aware of our centre of gravity, which is the belly, or *hara* (see p.51). If we ensure that our movements originate from our *hara*, then they will involve our whole body, thereby utilizing the sum total of our body's power. More specifically, all movement should originate from a point within the *hara* found just below the navel. This is our central pivotal point and is known as the *tanden* – the focal point of the *hara*.

If you watch babies move, it is very clear that their movements originate from their centre, their belly. You never see young babies tensing in the shoulder to push a toy. If you can get a baby to crawl on your back, you will experience the key qualities of shiatsu contact: complete surrender of weight to gravity, movements and balance, centred on and emanating from the belly.

Posture

Maintaining correct posture while giving shiatsu will make it easier for you to support the receiver's body without becoming tired, and will help you to move around their body more efficiently. This, in turn, helps your own Ki to flow smoothly around your body. The basic rules of good shiatsu posture are:

- Adopt a wide base with your legs, to ensure you maintain a low centre of gravity.

- Keep your *hara* relaxed and open.
- Look ahead, not down at the receiver (although check occasionally to see if the receiver is comfortable).
- Keep your shoulders relaxed.
- Keep your chest open, without forcing it.
- Keep the back of your neck lengthening and relaxed.
- Imagine that the spaces within the joints of your spine, shoulder, elbows, wrist and fingers are constantly opening as they become more relaxed.

How to position your body correctly

When giving shiatsu make sure that your *hara* is aligned with the area upon which you are working; or to get as close to that ideal as is practical without sacrificing your comfort. If you relax your body when applying pressure, your position will enable more of your body-weight to manifest onto the area you are working. The more your *hara* is aligned with your direction of pressure, the more your Ki will connect with the receiver. Connecting your Ki simply means aligning your intention with your action, or taking the most direct route to accomplish your goal. For example, when you are hungry, you turn to face the food cupboard and walk directly toward it. You do not walk sideways or backward. Your *hara* points the way. The urge to eat is your intention. Your mind maps out the route to the food, and your *hara* follows it. First you had the idea; the mind then led your Ki toward its goal; your Ki then enabled you to fulfil your goal.

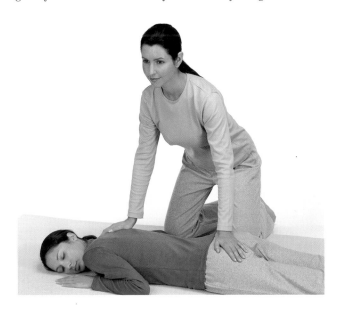

TECHNIQUE APPLICATION

We have established how and why we should prepare our body and mind to give shiatsu, and covered some basic background theory, so we can now explore how to apply some classical shiatsu techniques. These techniques employ various parts of the body. The most used tools are the palms, fingers and thumbs, but we can also use forearms, elbows, knees and feet to good effect. Shiatsu technique can be divided into three general categories: tonification, dispersal and calming. Using techniques from each of these categories has different aims and will have different effects on the receiver.

Tonification is used to build up areas of weak Ki (known as *kyo*) and is achieved by applying sustained pressure at the correct angle to reach deep into the pressure points, or *tsubos*, of the body. This increases the level of energy and blood circulating through that area, and boosts the channels suffering from *kyo*. Dispersal (sometimes called sedation) is achieved by using active techniques such as shaking, rocking, stretching, circling and squeezing, and is used to clear away blocked or congested energy and blood. Calming technique consists of lightly holding parts of the receiver's body with the palm of the hand or very gently rocking these areas, to calm agitated energy. A practitioner will usually employ all three of these methods during a shiatsu session, with a bias toward one or other depending upon the predominant type of energetic imbalance as assessed by the practitioner at the beginning of the session.

Palms

The palms are the main application tool used in basic-level shiatsu. Although less specific than using the thumbs or fingertips, the palms have a more soothing quality for the receiver. They are also icons of interpersonal communication, as shown by the common gesture of shaking the hand of someone you meet.

When performing shiatsu your palms and fingers must remain relaxed, with the whole surface of your palm in full contact with the recipient. Allow your hands to mould around the contours of their body, so that the palms lie quite flat when in contact with the back, or curl to envelop a more curved surface, such as an arm or the head. Your arms should be outstretched, but with the elbows unlocked. When you require closer body contact, you may need to have your arms at a 90-degree angle at the elbow, with the knee or inner thigh supporting your upper arm. Note, this will cause a slight reduction in the connection of Ki flow between your *hara* and your palm.

The following images show some of the most common shiatsu techniques using the palms.

1   **Support hand technique** Keep both hands separated but in contact with the receiver. This is the most basic, yet most important therapeutic shiatsu technique. It enables us to "listen" with one hand while the other hand is engaged in techniques to tonify, calm or disperse Ki. The "listening" hand is often called the support hand or mother hand. The active hand is sometimes called the working hand or child hand.

2   **Palm overlap technique** Place one hand on top of the other. This technique can be used when a malleable

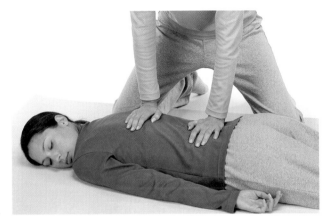

1

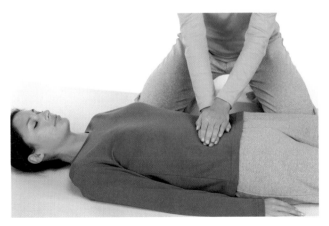

2

"wave like" action is required. It is often used directly on the receiver's belly for dispersing blocked Ki.

3 **Circular rotations** With one palm moulded into the contours of the shoulder blade, buttocks or lower back, rotate the connective tissues over the underlying bone rather than merely scrubbing the surface. The other palm can be positioned either nearby on the body, or on top of the first hand. Circular rotations are particularly effective for relieving muscular tensions around the shoulder blades. They also help to stimulate warmth in the pelvic region.

4 **Grasping** Use one hand to clasp the arm or leg for support, while moving the other along the limb squeezing gently. Also, while in this position you can use both hands to clasp a limb as you stretch that limb away from the space between your hands.

5 **Double palm squeezing** Interlock your fingers and apply a squeezing movement simultaneously with the heels of both hands. Double palm squeezing is useful for compressing the muscles either side of the lumbar spine – the area located between the kidneys and the pelvis.

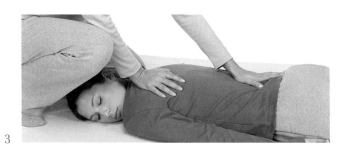

3

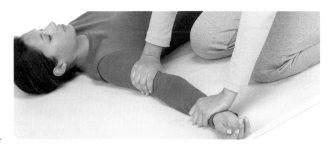

4

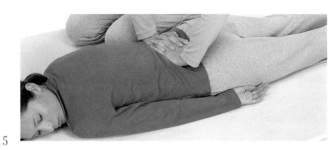

5

Adopt the pace of nature: her secret is patience.

RALPH WALDO EMERSON

(1803–1882)

A bird does not sing because it has an answer.
It sings because it has a song.

CHINESE PROVERB

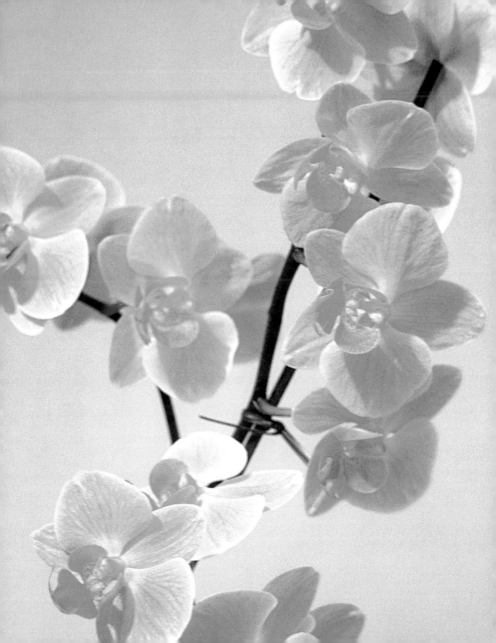

Thumbs

The thumb is the classic tool of shiatsu, and enables you
to apply stronger pressure than that exercised by the
fingers alone. Generally you should use the ball of the
thumb, but you can employ the area closer to the tip if
you require lighter pressure such as may be needed for
work on the face or the neck.

You may find that you have difficulty keeping your
thumbs straight, allowing them to buckle at the inter-
phalangeal joint. Try to avoid this because if you apply
strong pressure with buckled thumbs over a period of
time you will damage your thumb joints. Do not apply
even light pressure with buckled thumbs. There are two
main methods for supporting your thumb pressure – the
open hand and the closed hand methods.

1 **Open hand method** For maximum stability place your
   thumb in contact with the receiver's body and your other
   four fingers spread out and lightly touching the body.
2 **Closed hand method** Use your four fingers to form a
   fist, supporting your thumb against your index finger.

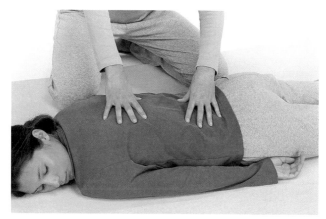

1

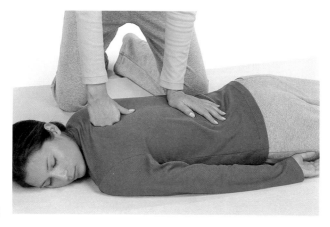

2

Fingers

The fingertips are excellent tools for sensing the Ki within the channels and for feeling other subtle activity registering near the surface of the receiver's body. This is because they have such a rich supply of sensory nerve endings. Make sure you keep your fingernails and thumbnails short. Nails have no sensory nerve endings, so you will feel nothing through them. However, the receiver will certainly feel something if you dig your nails into their body!

The following images show some of the most common shiatsu techniques using the fingers.

1 **Three or four finger method** Use the middle three fingers simultaneously to track along a Ki channel to find the discrepancies of Ki level within it. This is also an excellent technique for tonifying the spaces between the ribs, close to the breastbone. Place all four fingers of one hand on the receiver's mid- or upper back and circle or shake them for an effective method to disperse tension in the intercostal muscles between the ribs.

A two-handed version of this technique can be used to disperse tension in the muscles close to the spine, using a "push-pull" movement. For this technique your thumb should be relaxed and your fingers strong. Like all shiatsu techniques, the movement must originate from your *hara*, with a sense of connection to *tanden* (see p.55). This will prevent fatigue and tension accumulating in your wrist.

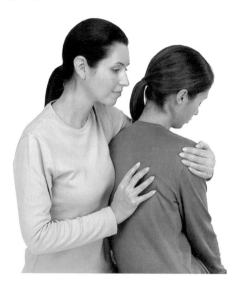

1

2 **Index finger method** This technique offers a useful alternative to the thumbs for practitioners who have hypermobile thumb joints. This is because the index finger is supported by the middle finger, thus making it very stable. It is a particularly useful technique for applying pressure to the side of the nose.

3 **"Vee" finger method** To employ this technique the middle and index fingers are lightly pressed either side of the spinal column or around the shoulder area simultaneously. It is mostly used on very small children,

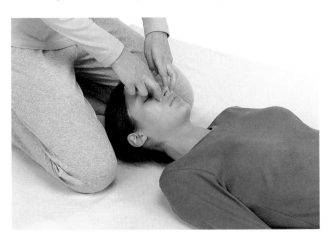

2

because the *tsubos* in a small back are far too small to accommodate shiatsu-level pressure from the thumbs.

Experienced shiatsu practitioners employ various combinations of techniques using their thumbs and fingers simultaneously for an advanced level of shiatsu work, but the methods shown on the preceeding pages are appropriate for beginner-level shiatsu, that is intended primarily to facilitate relaxation and reduce everyday stress.

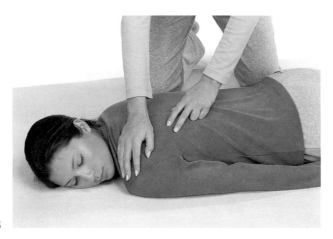

3

Forearms

Use the area of your forearm close to your elbow to apply strong pressure to the back, hips and feet. Apply the forearm, or both forearms together, only after you have warmed up the area to be worked by shiatsu techniques using your hands. This is because the hands are much more sensitive than the forearms and, as such, are by far the better tools with which to "read" a receiver's body and assess their Ki levels.

There are two basic methods for applying pressure to the receiver with your forearms, illustrated opposite on the sole of the foot and on the back.

1 **Single forearm technique** If you apply one forearm to the sole of the foot it gives a great feeling of ironing out tension in that area. Make sure your wrist is totally relaxed. Remember that all the pressure must come from leaning on, and not pushing, the receiver.

2 **Double forearm technique** Use both forearms together on the back, to give it a good stretch. You can also employ this method on the buttocks or thighs.

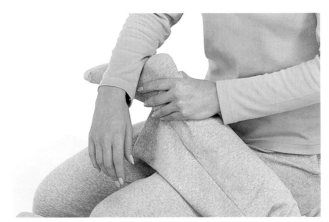

1

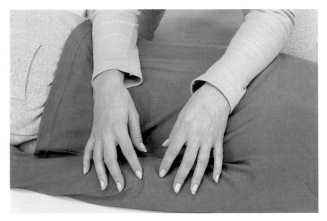

2

Elbows and knees

You can use both the elbows and the knees in shiatsu to apply firm pressure to the receiver's body. Adjust the level of this pressure to suit both your level of experience and the comfort of the receiver.

1   **Elbow technique** Elbows are useful when you require a strong, focused pressure. An elbow that is acutely flexed will provide the strongest pressure, but this can be excessive for many people. However, you can apply a

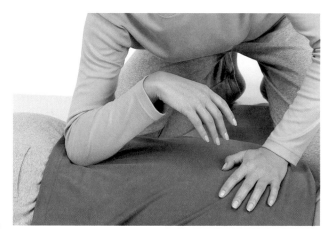

1

more comfortable pressure when the angle of the elbow is more open. It is essential to keep the wrist relaxed and the fist open, as this will prevent tension from building up in your arm.

2   **Knee technique** You can apply very firm pressure with your knees, and can develop great "knee sensitivity" by practising advanced techniques with them, but they will never be as sensitive as your hands. As such you should use them with discretion and only on areas previously checked by your hands. Apply your knees together or

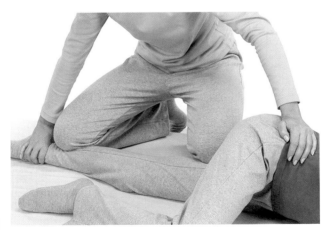

2

individually. Keep both hands on the receiver's body while you are working with your knees so that your body-weight is supported through your hands rather than through your knees. Your hands must be positioned so that you can instantly remove your knees if necessary, to ensure the receiver's comfort and your own stability.

Feet

You can use your feet to a lesser or greater extent depending on the style of shiatsu (see pp.16–17) you

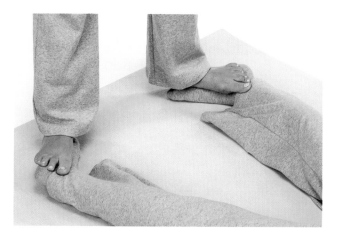

practise. They are less sensitive than the hands, but are useful for applying strong pressure. Also, because they spend most of their time directly against the ground, they bring an "earthy" quality to the session. Regularly walking around in bare feet will enhance this earthy, grounded quality in your shiatsu work.

Use the feet to stand on the receiver's feet to ground them (opposite). Alternatively use them to temporarily disperse blocked Ki in the limbs via a rapid shaking technique (below), applied with light pressure.

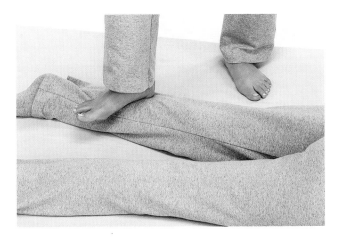

Stretching

As well as using hands, knees, feet and elbows to apply direct pressure within shiatsu technique, you can also apply a direct therapeutic stretch to various parts of the receiver's body to help balance their Ki. Accurate and appropriate stretching requires as much sensitivity as applying pressure, but practising and developing a good stretching technique will enable you to achieve many benefits for your recipient in a relatively short time.

Stretching (sometimes also called "opening") is a useful part of shiatsu for many reasons. It can improve general flexibility and ease muscular tension. It also supports the blood and lymphatic circulatory systems and can improve respiration by helping to open up the ribcage. Perhaps most importantly, stretching can bring the Ki channels closer to the surface so that they can be accessed more easily, and can help disperse blocked Ki.

Actually, you are not really "stretching" the muscle or a limb by this work, rather you help it to relax more, so that it lengthens by way of letting go of residual tension. In shiatsu practice there are three types of stretching:

1 **Gravity stretching** With this type of shiatsu stretch the pratitioner places the recipient in a position that enables gravity to "open" the limb being worked on as they allow themselves to let go and surrender to its forces. This requires no further intervention by the practitioner other than to steady the limb if required.

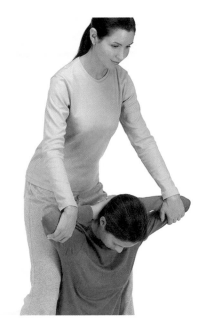

1

2 **Passive-assisted stretch** Move the receiver's limb slowly until it reaches its maximum "open" position. This is similar to gravity stretching except that as the practitioner you are adopting the role of gravity. It is more effective than gravity stretching because you can encourage a greater stretch in the receiver by adding a little bit of extra movement.

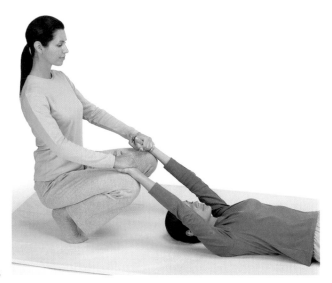

2

3 **Facilitated stretch** With this type of stretch you initially ask the recipient to push their limb, against resistance, away from the direction in which you ultimately want them to stretch. Then move the limb in the opposite direction into its maximum open position. By contracting the muscle before giving it a passive-assisted stretch, you achieve a greater stretch on the limb.

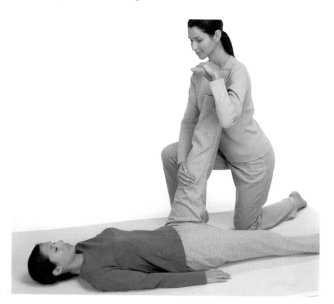

3

Greatness lies not in being strong,
but in the correct use of strength.

HENRY WARD BEECHER

(1813–1887)

If a person concentrates on one thing and does not get
away from it ... he will possess strong, moving power.

CHENG YI

(1033–1107)

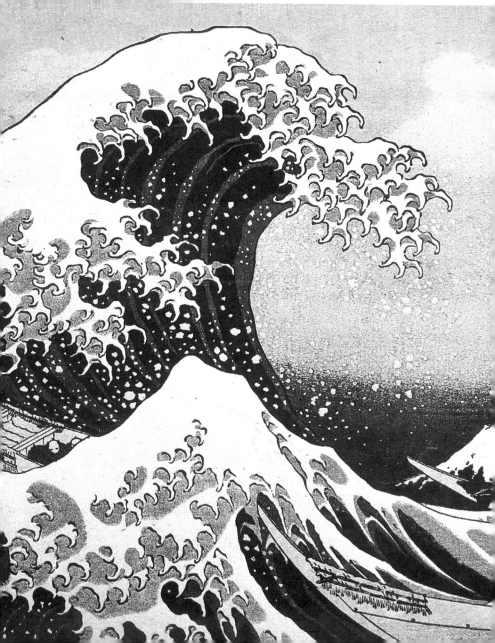

Chapter Four

basic shiatsu sequences

We are now at the stage where we can look at how
specific shiatsu techniques can be linked together to
produce technical sequences. Such sequences, or
"forms" as they are sometimes called, occur with the
recipient placed in a variety of possible positions. The
most popular of these are: receiver face down, receiver face up, and receiver lying on his or her side.
Having the receiver sitting upright on the floor or on
a chair can also be useful, but it is less commonly
practised than the other positions, because most people prefer to lie down to receive treatment as this is
generally more relaxing. A short sequence in each of
these positions is described in the following pages.

Some specific techniques applied to the *hara* (belly) and chest are also included as a separate sequence, because working on the *hara* is the main focus of some traditional Japanese shiatsu styles.

Please note that these sequences are not intended as a "teach yourself" manual, and are no substitute for professional training. Shiatsu has many complex nuances which require in-class tuition and close supervision to master. Rather, we reprise here some of the basic techniques that you would expect to learn in a shiatsu class. If you would like to practice shiatsu for general interest or with a view to becoming a professional therapist, it is imperative that you train at a reputable shiatsu school (see p.128).

FACE-DOWN SEQUENCE

Before you begin working on a receiver who is lying in the face-down position, check that he or she is relaxed and comfortable (this applies to all of the shiatsu sequences presented in this chapter). If necessary, place small cushions under each of the receiver's ankles to help relax their legs. If possible, get them to rest their arms on the floor by their sides, as this will make it easier for you to work on the upper back. However, if the receiver is significantly more comfortable with their arms on the floor beyond their head, you should allow this. The aim is to make them as comfortable as possible in order to facilitate their total relaxation so that they will gain maximum benefit from the shiatsu session.

Begin by placing both your hands on the receiver's back. Remember to look ahead, not down, and to focus your attention on the present moment. Become aware of the receiver's breathing. You will feel this via the gentle rising and falling of their ribs. Once you have checked your own posture you are ready to start.

1 **Baby walking** Kneel beside the recipient with your knees spread to ensure a solid base from which to apply the technique. Keep your head up and your *hara* relaxed and open. Lean your bodyweight through your hands and "walk" your hands randomly over the receiver's back and buttocks; just like a baby crawling. Allow gravity to determine the level of pressure rather than applying pressure through pushing. Take care when working on the lower back and spinal column. This technique will have a relaxing effect on the receiver.

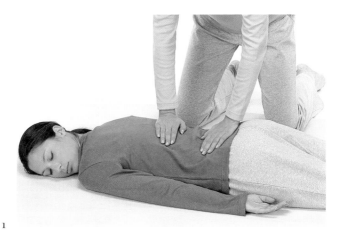

1

2 **Stretching muscles away from the upper spine** This technique eliminates upper-back stiffness. From a kneeling or squatting position, place both hands on the far side of the receiver's upper back, with the heel of the hands in the natural groove close to their spine. Allow your body-weight to fall into the receiver's back through the heels of both hands equally, thus gently stretching the muscles away from their spine. Move to the opposite side of the receiver's body and repeat the technique on the other side of the spine.

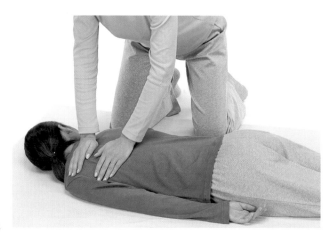

2

3 **Open diagonal stretch** Position one palm on the near side of the receiver's upper back, with the heel of your hand close to the inside edge of their shoulderblade. Put your other hand on their far side buttock so that your hands are positioned diagonally. Lean your *hara* forward toward the space between your two hands and feel your hands splay apart. Let this effect take up the slack in their skin, thus giving them a diagonal stretch across their entire back. Keep your shoulders down, your belly relaxed and your head up. Repeat on the opposite side.

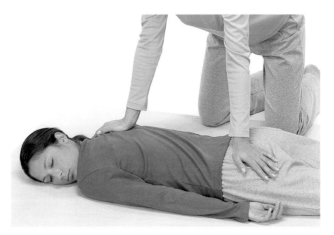

3

4 **Open longitudinal back stretch** The method for this
   stretch is the same as for the open diagonal stretch (see
   p.89) except that you place both hands on the same side
   of the body. This will "open" one side of the back at a
   time, in a longitudinal direction, rather than diagonally.
   Take care when performing this technique with the
   hands on the near side of the receiver's back as it can be
   easy to let yourself become slightly hunched over. These
   back stretches can help alleviate lower backache as a
   result of stress or poor posture.

5 **Crossed-arm backstretch** The open diagonal and open
   longitudinal stretches (3 and 4) can also be applied by
   crossing your arms, as with this stretch. Here, place the
   upper hand much lower on the receiver's back, on the
   lower ribs. This isolates the stretch to the lumbar region
   only. It is a good option when working on somebody
   much smaller than yourself, because it enables you to
   spread your hands away from one another as you stretch.
   When the hands are too close together, as might be the
   case on a smaller client, it is much more difficult to get
   the hands to stretch open if they are not crossed.

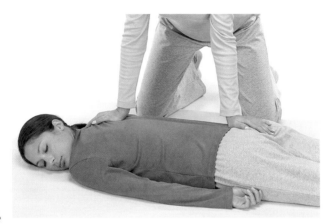

4

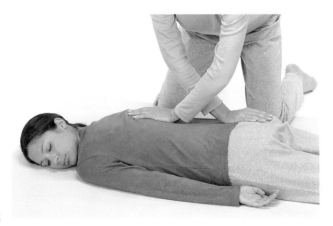

5

6 **Forearm back stretch** You can also perform the open diagonal and open longitudinal stretches to the back using the underside of your forearms as opposed to your hands. Keep your wrists totally flaccid and, if necessary, move your knees a little further away from the receiver's body, to allow yourself sufficient room to relax your *hara*. Although your posture will be much lower to the ground in this method, try to resist the temptation to look down at the receiver – instead look ahead, empty your mind and focus on the present moment.

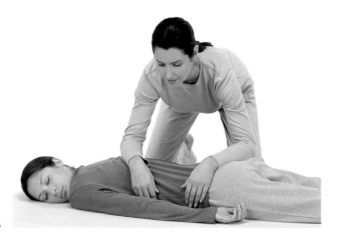

6

7 **Thumbs down back** Position yourself at the head of the receiver, facing toward their feet. Locate the bony protrusions of the spinal column. Starting in the upper back below the base of the neck, glide your thumbs either side of the spine to a position about one-and-a-half thumb-widths lateral to the vertebral column. Lean in with your thumbs so that the angle of pressure is at right angles to the contour of the back. Use your body weight, not strength. Check with the receiver that you are not causing them any pain. Withdraw your thumbs and glide

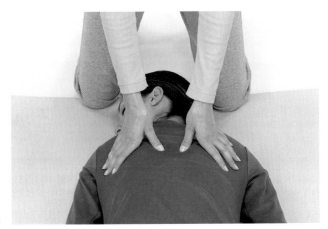

7

93

them adjacent to the space between the next vertebrae. Continue working down the spine until you reach the middle of the back. Then glide your hands back to just below the base of the neck and repeat.

8 **Palm down back of legs** Kneel beside the receiver with one knee adjacent to their hip and the other knee next to their upper leg. Place your support hand on the sacrum and use your other hand to palm down the back of the thigh to the knee. Avoid leaning pressure into the back of the knee, although you can make a light connection there with your palm. Now move your position closer to their feet so that your support hand rests on their lower thigh. Palm down toward the heels. Do not lean excessive pressure into the calf as it is often a tender area.

9 **Forearm into sole of foot** Place the receiver's foot on your thigh so that the shape of their ankle and foot fits precisely into the contour of your thigh. Your other knee should rest on the back of their thigh or on the floor. Lean your forearm into the sole of their foot, keeping your wrist fully relaxed.

Repeat techniques 8 and 9 on the other leg.

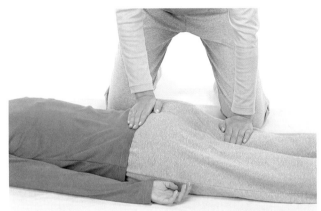

8

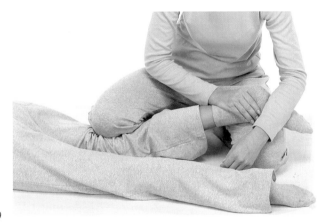

9

FACE-UP SEQUENCE

Invite the receiver to lie on their back and make sure that they are comfortable. Place a pillow under their head if desired. Before you begin to perform any shiatsu techniques on someone lying in the face-up position, spend a minute or two kneeling next to them with one hand resting on their *hara* and your other hand holding their wrist or hand. This will help to create a particular attunement between the two of you.

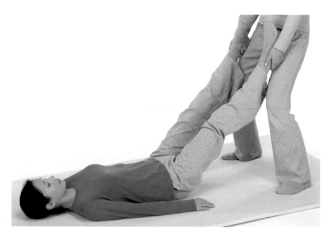

1

1 **Pulling heels** Stand at the receiver's feet, facing their head. Place your hands under their heels and pick up the feet. Lift the heels high enough for their lower back to flatten against the floor. Lean back until you see their chin move slightly toward the chest, indicating that their spine is being lengthened a little.

2 **Hip circling** Kneel to the side of one of the receiver's hips. Hold their knee with one hand and their heel with the other. Bend their knee toward their chest. Draw outward circles in the air with their leg.

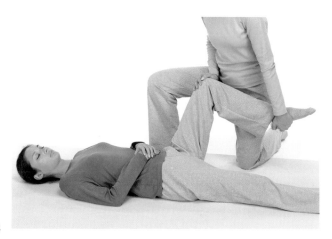

2

3   **Single knee to chest** After performing the hip-circling technique, move it into this technique by leaning some of your weight toward the receiver's chest. Keep your head up and avoid looking down at the receiver's face when their knee is pressed close to their chest, as this might startle them if they open their eyes. Together, these two techniques will relax and open the hips.

4   **Foot to *hara*** Support the receiver's leg as you straighten it, and position yourself in a wide, kneeling stance so that the outside edge of their foot rests squarely in your

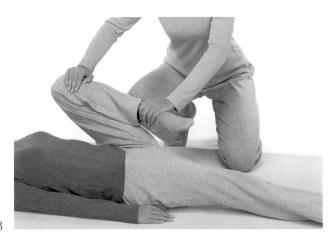

3

hara, embraced by your two hands. Lean your *hara* into their foot and circle the foot using your whole body. If they have hyper-extended knees (knees that bend the wrong way slightly), or experience discomfort in the knee during this technique, use one hand or some cushions to support the back of their knee; thus keeping it unlocked. This technique will calm the receiver and will also help to ground them at the same time.

Repeat techniques 2 to 4 on the other leg, trying not to break contact as you take your time moving across.

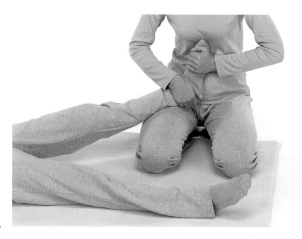

4

5   **Palming down arm** Lay the receiver's arm on the
    ground at right angles to their torso and position your-
    self against their side, facing away from their feet. Palm
    along the arm, starting close to the shoulder and moving
    outward toward their wrist. Keep the hand that is closer
    to their shoulder stationary while your other hand palms
    down toward the elbow. Once past the elbow, one of your
    hands should remain stationary close to the elbow while
    your other hand palms down toward the hand. When you
    apply pressure through both palms, try to do it equally.

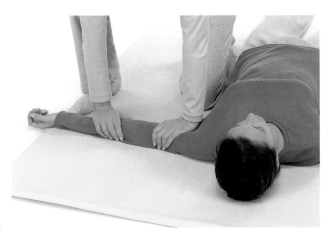

5

6   **Hand to *hara*** Position yourself at the receiver's head facing their feet. Adopt a wide kneeling position. Bring one of their arms on to your thigh and hold the back of their hand against your *hara*. If you have their left hand in your *hara*, you should be holding it with your right hand, and vice versa. Rest your other hand on their armpit or upper arm, then slowly lean gentle pressure through your hand along their arm toward their elbow.

Repeat techniques 5 and 6 on the other arm. Replace the arm on the ground by the receiver's side to conclude.

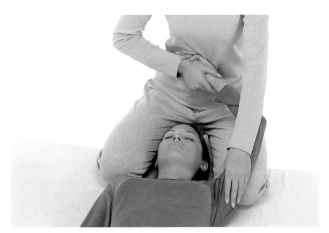

6

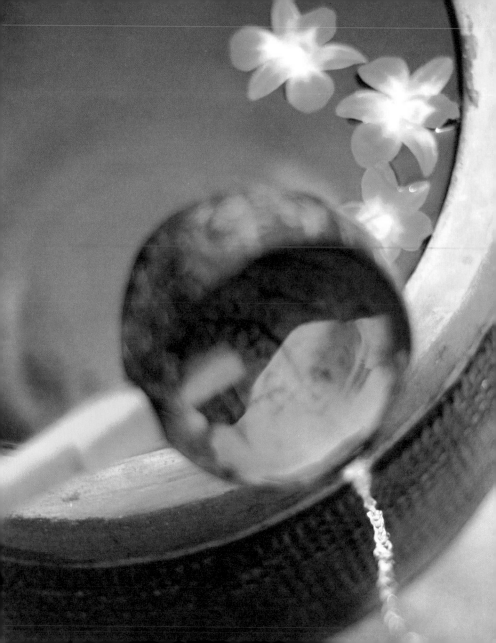

When an ordinary man attains knowledge,
he is a sage; when a sage attains understanding,
he is an ordinary man.

ZEN PROVERB

LYING-ON-SIDE SEQUENCE

Shiatsu given in the side position has certain advantages over shiatsu in the prone (face-down) or supine (face-up) position as it enables full mobility of the shoulders, arms, hips and legs, and allows greater movement of the torso. Also, people with back problems often find it difficult to relax fully in any position other than this one. This sequence concentrates mainly on the shoulder and arm. To ensure the receiver is comfortable in this position, place some padding under their head and knee.

1 **Trapezius stretch** Kneel next to the receiver, in contact with their body and facing toward their head. Place their uppermost forearm over your closest forearm so that their arm does not drag on the floor. Clasping your hands around their shoulder, lean back using your body weight to "open" their neck. If their head comes away from the pillow, you have leaned back too strongly.

2 **Shoulder girdle rotation** From the trapezius stretch, rotate the receiver's shoulder girdle in an "up, back and

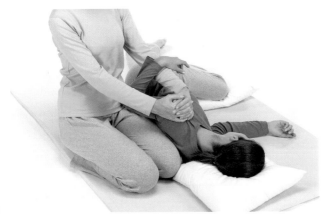

1

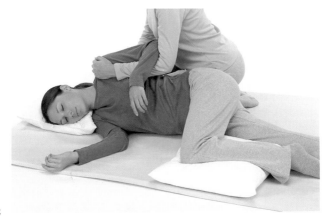

2

down" direction, to encourage their chest to open. Your whole body should be involved in the rotation, not just your arms. Alternate between the trapezius stretch and shoulder girdle rotation for one or two minutes. These techniques will help release any stress-induced tension in the receiver's neck and shoulders.

3 **Vertical arm stretch** From shoulder girdle rotation remove one hand from the receiver's shoulder and use it to clasp their uppermost hand or wrist. Place your other hand on their upper arm and swivel up into a half kneel-

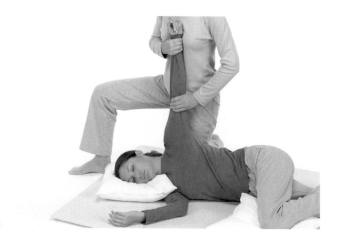

3

ing position to face the same direction as they are facing. Sink down a little and embrace their arm, giving it as much contact as possible with your arms and torso. Straighten and lengthen your posture. This will result in a traction of their shoulder girdle, shoulder, elbow and wrist joints. This stretch will also benefit their heart.

4 **Lance stretch** Next circle the receiver's arm to a position whereby it is projecting beyond their head, so that you are moving toward creating a straight line between their upper hip, shoulder and hand. Keep your hands in

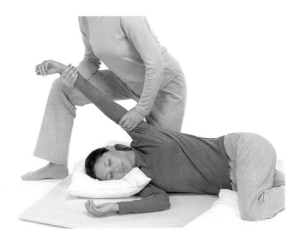

4

the same position as in the vertical arm stretch, and rest your forearm on your knee. Lean away from their feet. This opens the side of their ribs and aids liver function.

5   **Side torso gall bladder stretch** Place the receiver's hand on the floor beyond their head. If their shoulder joint lacks full mobility, you can place their arm in front of their chest instead. Kneel behind them midway between their hip and shoulder. Cross your arms and place one hand on their hip and the other hand on the lower ribs. Lean down and open their waist area. Make sure that you do not lean into the armpit area, as this will cause pain there and discomfort to their neck and shoulder. This technique greatly benefits the liver and gall bladder functions.

6   **Arm to body stretch** Place the receiver's arm against their body. Put a cushion between their arm and their waist to avoid stressing their elbow joint. Lean your palms or thumbs in a travelling movement along the arm and wrist. Do not lean too strongly into their shoulder area, as this may cause discomfort to the neck. This technique benefits the bowels and intestines.

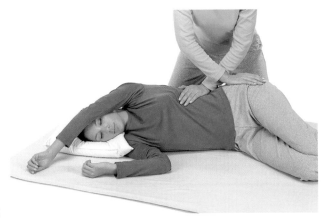

5

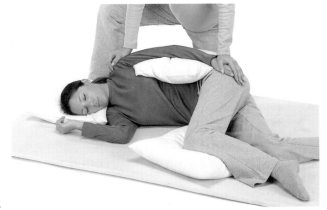

6

SITTING SEQUENCE

Applying shiatsu to a receiver in the sitting position has the advantage of enabling you to move their torso in any direction – a situation that does not exist in any of the other positions. The shoulder and neck are also more accessible and mobile. Also, this is a good position if you want to encourage the receiver to stay more alert during the session than they might otherwise do if lying down. In many sitting techniques the receiver has to maintain his or her own upright posture. Because of this it is rare for a them to doze off in this position!

Invite the receiver either to kneel on the floor or to sit with crossed legs. Many people will find that the crossed-leg position is more comfortable. Also, it may be easier for them to remain fully upright in this position if they sit with buttocks raised up on a firm cushion or a foam block 5–6cm (2–2⅓in) thick. If your intended receiver is not comfortable or able to sit in either position, you can perform many of the following techniques with them sitting on a stool.

1 **Palming down spine** Kneel an arms-length distance behind the receiver. Place a support hand on their shoulder, close to the base of their neck. Leaning from your *hara*, use your other hand to palm down their back; either over their spine or to the side of the spine (the same side as the shoulder held by your support hand). Take care not to push them forward. Repeat on the other side, placing your support hand on their other shoulder.

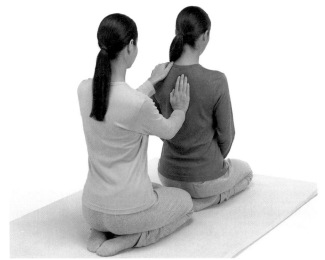

1

2 **Arm circling** Position yourself beside and slightly behind the receiver, and place your support hand over their shoulder. Now cradle their arm in your arm and rotate it backward in a motion resembling the back-stroke arm movement. This mobilizes the shoulder and benefits the lungs and intestines. Repeat this movement on the other arm.

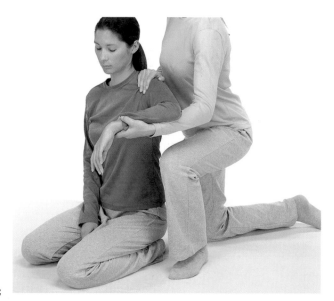

2

3 **Single arm overhead stretch** Progressing directly from
   arm circling, keep the same arm cradled in your arm and
   place your support hand on their other shoulder. Bring
   the arm over their head, thus giving their inner arm and
   armpit a mild opening stretch. This will benefit the
   heart by opening the heart channel. Keep your thigh in
   close contact with their torso to support this position.

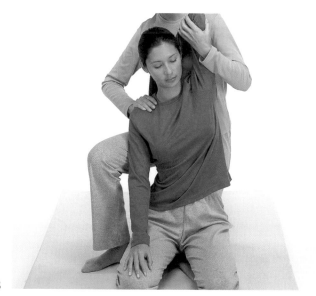

3

4   **Child pose low back stretch** Invite the receiver to kneel with their head resting on the floor or on a cushion. From a standing position place one hand on one side of their lumbar area and the other hand on the opposite hip. Apply a diagonal stretch. Avoid leaning too high up their back because this will compress their neck and squash their face into the floor. This is a good technique to help alleviate a stiff lower back.

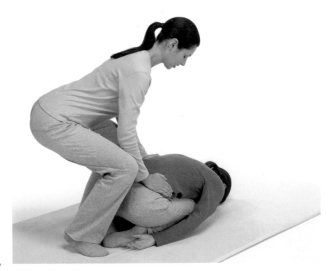

4

5 **Thumbs into lower back** Continuing from technique 4, carefully lean your thumbs into the receiver's lower back a couple of thumb-widths either side of the spine, and move progressively from the waistline down into the bony sacrum of their buttocks. Afterward, help the receiver to sit back up. They will be very relaxed after receiving these techniques, so make sure they sit up slowly to avoid feeling dizzy.

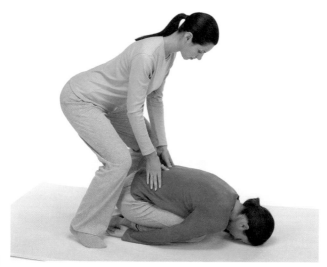

5

HARA AND CHEST SEQUENCE

In contrast to the back, which is a tough and relatively hard area, the *hara* and chest are sensitive, vulnerable parts of the body that we instinctively want to protect, and some people may feel nervous or unsure about receiving treatment to this area. Consequently, it is important to gain the receiver's confidence and trust before applying any shiatsu techniques here.

For techniques applied directly on to the *hara*, the practitioner should be positioned on the right-hand side of the receiver. The reason for this is that techniques applied to this area from the direction of the right can greatly facilitate bowel movement. (This is because the colon rises on the right hand side, crosses from right to left, and descends down the left side of the belly into the anus.) If any of the following techniques cause pain or nausea for the receiver, then you should stop immediately. Also, avoid giving shiatsu soon after the receiver has eaten, and never apply shiatsu to this area if the receiver is pregnant.

1 **Wave rocking** Kneel down facing toward the receiver's *hara*. Place one of your hands on top of the other and rhythmically knead the belly with a motion similar to that of a wave breaking upon the shore. Try not to move your hands too quickly, as this can cause the receiver to feel nauseous (it makes them literally seasick). Instead imagine you are on the beach at the edge of a calm sea, and time your movements to synchronize with the wavelets in the sea that you observe breaking gently upon the shore.

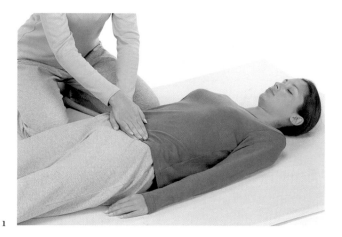

1

2 **Bowl rotations** Form an inverted bowl shape with both hands and place the centre of the bowl over the receiver's belly. Now slowly rotate the bowl's rim around the belly, upon a central axis, in a clockwise direction. The reason you move clockwise is to conform to the direction of the bowel movement. This technique will facilitate the receiver's bowel movement and help to ease any constipation. Conversely, moving in a counter-clockwise direction may inhibit such movement. Remember to keep the pace gentle.

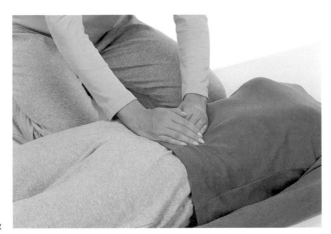

2

3 **Bowl circling** This technique shares the same hand position as bowl rotations, but you should move the bowl around the receiver's body in a clockwise direction, as if you are stirring a big pot of porridge with both hands, thereby stretching the soft tissues of the belly more. This is a helpful technique for aiding sluggish bowels and poor circulation in the abdomen. Bowl circling and bowl rotations can be performed alternately – doing so offers the added bonus of providing good training for your own coordination.

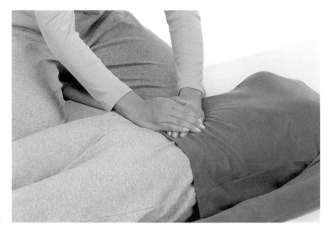

3

4 **Gathering to the centre** Gather the receiver's flesh from varying directions toward the navel with both of your hands, but generally progressing in a clockwise direction. This increases blood circulation to the intestines and the muscles deep within the belly. If you cannot pick up the flesh because it is too tight, ask the receiver to bend their legs so their knees are raised and the soles of the feet rest on the floor. You will then find the belly looser and easier to gather up. This is also the better leg position for anyone suffering lower back pain.

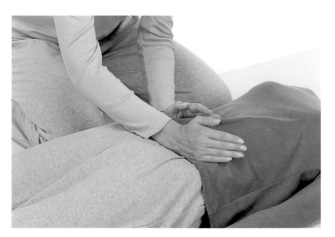

4

5   **Sternal cupping** Turn to face the receiver's head. Place the edges of both of your hands on either side of their breastbone and lean in very gently as the receiver exhales. As the centre of the chest, between the breasts, is an intimate area for a woman, it is better to explain what you intend to do before you do it, and then ask whether or not she minds if you proceed. This is especially important if you are a man working on a woman. This technique will help to regulate respiration and balance the functions of the kidneys and heart.

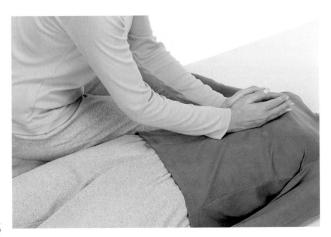

5

Balance is the perfect state of still water.
Let that be our model. It remains quiet within
and is not disturbed on the surface.

CONFUCIUS

(*c.*551–*c.*479BCE)

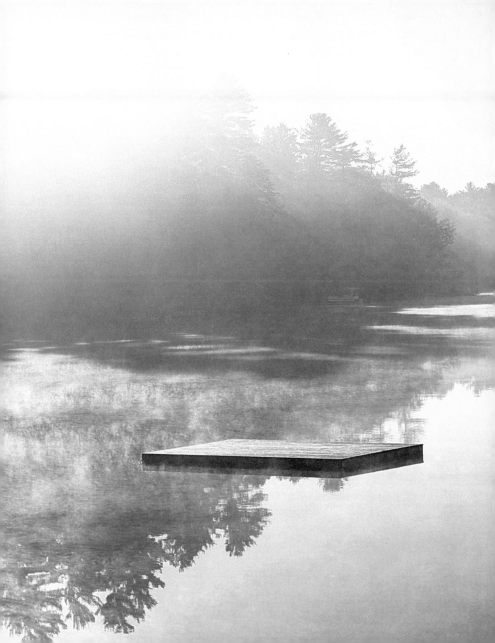

GLOSSARY

An Mo Traditional Chinese bodywork based on the principles of traditional Oriental medicine.

Anma Japanese bodywork method, based on *An Mo*, and a precursor of shiatsu.

Anma-Sotai An intermediate level of Japanese bodywork placed between basic-level and professional-level shiatsu.

Calming The shiatsu technique of lightly holding or gently rocking parts of the receiver's body in order to calm any agitated Ki.

Dispersal The shiatsu technique whereby a practitioner aims to address any *jitsu* in the receiver's Ki by applying active movements such as shaking, rocking and stretching to the affected areas.

"Empty-mind" state The intuitive, non-thinking state employed by a practitioner during a shiatsu session in order to best treat the receiver.

Hara The central pivotal area of the body, located in the belly, from which all shiatsu movements should begin.

Jitsu A state of fullness, stagnation or blockage in the flow of Ki around a person's body.

Ki The universal energy, present in all things, that flows around the body through interconnecting channels. Ki is manipulated by shiatsu treatment with the aim of optimizing the health and vitality of the receiver.

Kyo A state of weakness, emptiness or underactivity in the flow of Ki around a person's body.

Tanden Located just below the navel, the *tanden* is the focal point of the *hara* and the central pivotal point in the body.

Tonification The shiatsu technique whereby a practitioner aims to address any *kyo* in the receiver's Ki by applying sustained pressure to the *tsubos* on the body.

Tsubo A point on a Ki channel where the Ki can access or leave the body, and where a practitioner can assess the state of the flow of Ki around the receiver.

Yin and Yang The two opposite but complementary forces that co-exist in all things in the universe.

INDEX

PICTURE CREDITS / ACKNOWLEDGMENTS

Picture Credits

The publisher would like to thank the following people and photographic libraries for permission to reproduce their material. Every care has been taken to trace copyright holders. However, if we have omitted anyone we apologise and will, if informed, make corrections in any future editions.

Page 2 Getty/Image Bank/Ken Kochey; **18** Photos.com; **33** Photolibrary.com/Botanica/ Ann Cutting; **46** Photonica/Tatsuo Iizuka; **65** ZEFA/F Ruhe; **83** Art Archive/Claude Debussy Centre St Germain en Laye/Dagli Orti; **102** Photolibrary.com/Botanica/ Augustus Butera; **123** Getty/Image Bank/Ken Kochey

Publisher's Acknowledgments

Models: Caroline Long and Jasmine Hemsley
Make-up artist: Tinks Reding

Chris Jarmey runs The European Shiatsu School near Marlborough in Wiltshire. For information regarding shiatsu training courses run by the school, contact The European Shiatsu School, Central Administration, Highbank, Lockeridge, Marlborough, Wiltshire SN8 4EQ, UK; telephone: +44 (0) 1672 513444, email: info@shaitsu.net, websites: www.shiatsu.net and www.shiatsu.org.uk.